The Ultimate Air Fryer Guide for Meat Lovers

A Collection of Super Tasty Meat Based Recipes for Getting the Very Best Out of your New Air Fryer

By Donna Thomson

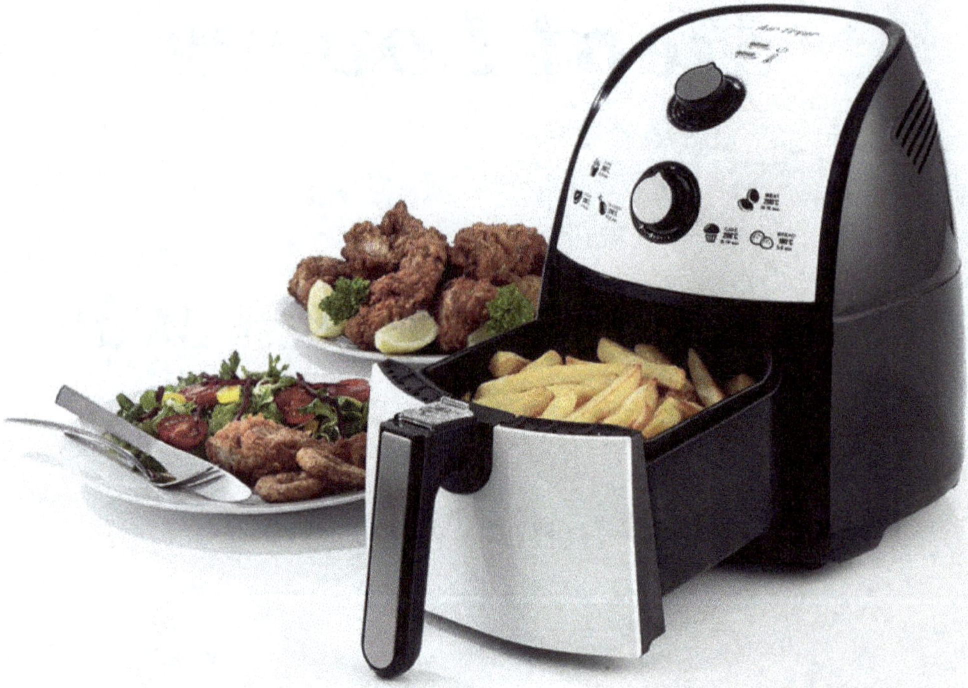

The content within this book has been derived from various sources. Please consult a licensed professional before attempting any techniques outlined in this book.

By reading this document, the reader agrees that under no circumstances is the author responsible for any losses, direct or indirect, which are incurred as a result of the use of information contained within this document, including, but not limited to, — errors, omissions, or inaccuracies

Table of Contents

Beef Brisket Recipe from Texas

Serves: 8

Cooking Time: one hour and 30 Minutes

Ingredients:

- 1 ½ cup beef stock /375ML
- 1 bay leaf
- 1 tablespoon garlic powder /15G
- 1 tablespoon onion powder /15G
- 2 pounds beef brisket, trimmed /900G
- 2 tablespoons chili powder /30G
- 2 teaspoons dry mustard /10G
- 4 tablespoons organic olive oil /60 ML
- Salt and pepper to taste

Instructions:

1) Preheat the air fryer for 5 minutes.
2) Place all ingredients in the deep baking pan.
3) Bake for an hour and 30 Minutes at 400° F or 205°C .
4) Stir the beef after every 30 minutes to allow the beef to soak in the sauce.

Nutrition information:

- Calories per serving: 306
- Carbohydrates: 3.8g

- Protein: 18.3g
- Fat: 24.1g

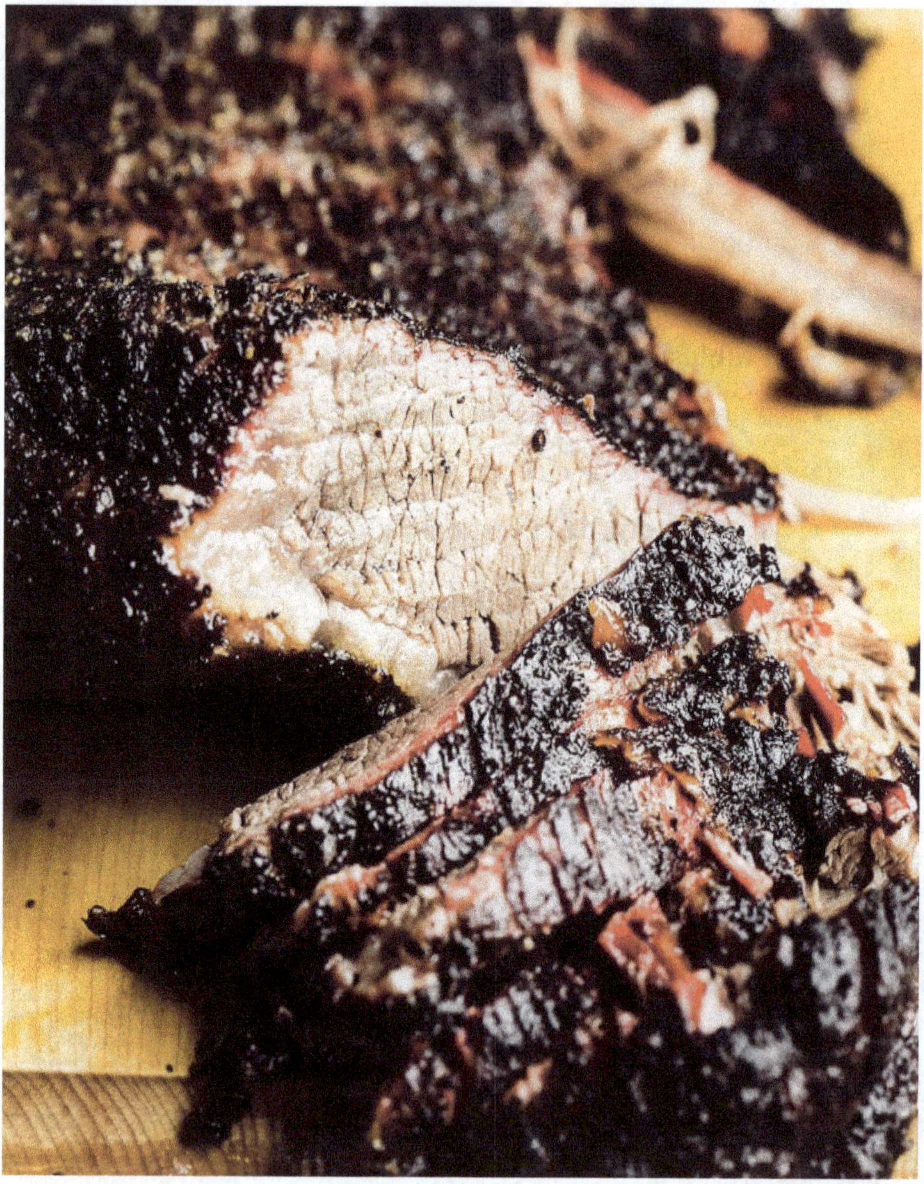

Beef Recipe Texas-Rodeo Style

Servings per Recipe: 6

Cooking Time: an hour

Ingredients:

- ½ cup honey /125ML
- ½ cup ketchup /125ML
- ½ teaspoon dry mustard /2.5G
- 1 clove of garlic, minced
- 1 tablespoon chili powder /15G
- 2 onion, chopped
- 3 pounds beef steak sliced /1350G
- Salt and pepper to taste

Instructions:

1) Place all ingredients in a Ziploc bag, place in the fridge and allow to marinate for about 120 minutes.
2) Preheat mid-air fryer to 390**O** F or 199°C .
3) Place the grill pan in the air fryer.
4) Grill the beef for 15 minutes per batch, turnover every 8 minutes for even grilling.
5) Meanwhile, pour the marinade over a saucepan and allow it to simmer over medium heat.
6) Baste the beef with sauce before serving.

Nutrition information:

- Calories per serving: 542
- Carbs: 49g
- Protein: 37g
- Fat: 22g

Beef Roast in Worcestershire-Rosemary

Serves: 6

Cooking Time: 2 hours

Ingredients:

- 1 onion, chopped
- 1 tablespoon butter /15G
- 1 tablespoon Worcestershire sauce /15ML
- 1 teaspoon rosemary /5G
- 1 teaspoon thyme /5G
- 1-pound beef chuck roast /450G
- 2 cloves of garlic, minced
- 2 tablespoons olive oil /30ML
- 3 cups water /750ML
- 3 stalks of celery, sliced

Instructions:

1) Preheat the air fryer for 5 minutes.
2) Place all ingredients in a deep baking dish that may fit into a mid-air fryer.
3) Bake for 120 minutes at 350° F or 177°C .
4) Steam the meat using its sauce, stir every 30 minutes until cooked.

Nutrition information:

- Calories per serving: 260
- Carbohydrates: 2.9g
- Protein: 17.5g
- Fat: 19.8

Beefy 'n Cheesy Spanish Rice Casserole

Servings per Recipe: 3

Cooking Time: 50 minutes

Ingredients:

- 2 tablespoons chopped green bell pepper /30G
- 1 tablespoon chopped fresh cilantro /15G
- 1/2-pound lean ground beef /225G
- 1/2 cup water /125ML
- 1/2 teaspoon salt /2.5G
- 1/2 teaspoon brown sugar /2.5G
- 1/2 pinch ground black pepper
- 1/3 cup uncooked long-grain rice /43G
- 1/4 cup finely chopped onion /32.5G
- 1/4 cup chile sauce /62.5ML
- 1/4 teaspoon ground cumin /1.25G
- 1/4 teaspoon Worcestershire sauce /1.25ML
- 1/4 cup shredded Cheddar cheese /32.5G
- 1/2 (14.5 ounces) can canned tomatoes /435G

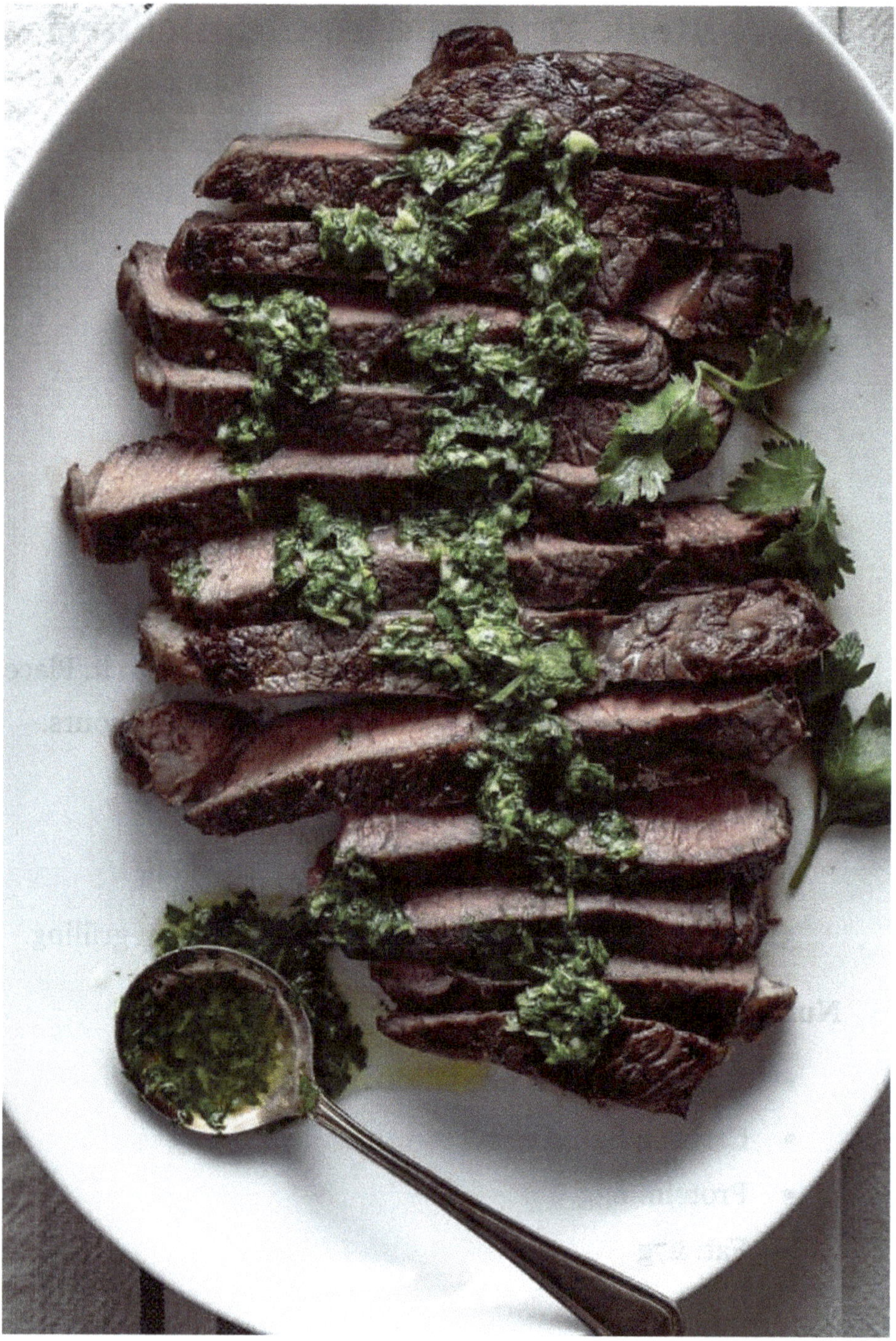

Bourbon-BBQ Sauce Marinated Beef BBQ

Servings per Recipe: 4

Cooking Time: 60 minutes

Ingredients:

- ¼ cup bourbon /62.5ML
- ¼ cup barbecue sauce /62.5ML
- 1 tablespoon Worcestershire sauce /15ML
- 2 pounds beef steak, pounded /900G
- Salt and pepper to taste

Instructions:

1) Place all ingredients in the Ziploc bag, place them in a fridge for a couple of hours to allow the ingredients to marinate.
2) Preheat the air fryer to 390 ° F or 199°C .
3) Place the grill pan accessory in the air fryer.
4) Place around the grill pan and cook for 20 minutes per batch.
5) Turnover and stir halfway the cooking time for even cooking.
6) Meanwhile, pour the marinade on the saucepan and allow it to simmer for 10 minutes
7) Serve beef with bourbon sauce.

- Carbs: 18.2g
- Protein: 24.4g
- Fat: 35.5g

Cajun Sweet-Sour Grilled Pork

Servings per Recipe: 3

Cooking Time: 12 minutes

Ingredients:

- ¼ cup brown sugar /32.5G
- 1/4 cup cider vinegar /62.5G
- 1-lb pork loin, sliced into 1-inch cubes /450G
- 2 tablespoons Cajun seasoning /30G
- 3 tablespoons brown sugar /45G

Instructions:

1) Mix the pork loin, 3 tablespoons brown sugar, and Cajun seasoning in a shallow bowl. Mix well to coat. Marinate in the refrigerator for 3 hours.
2) Mix brown sugar and vinegar in a shallow bowl for basting.
3) Thread pork pieces in skewers. Baste with sauce and place on a skewer rack in the air fryer.
4) Cook at 360° F or 183°C for 12 minutes, turn skewer halfway through cooking time and baste with sauce. If necessary, cook in batches.
5) Serve and enjoy

Nutrition Information:

- Calories per Serving: 428
- Carbs: 30.3g
- Protein: 39.0g
- Fat: 16.7g

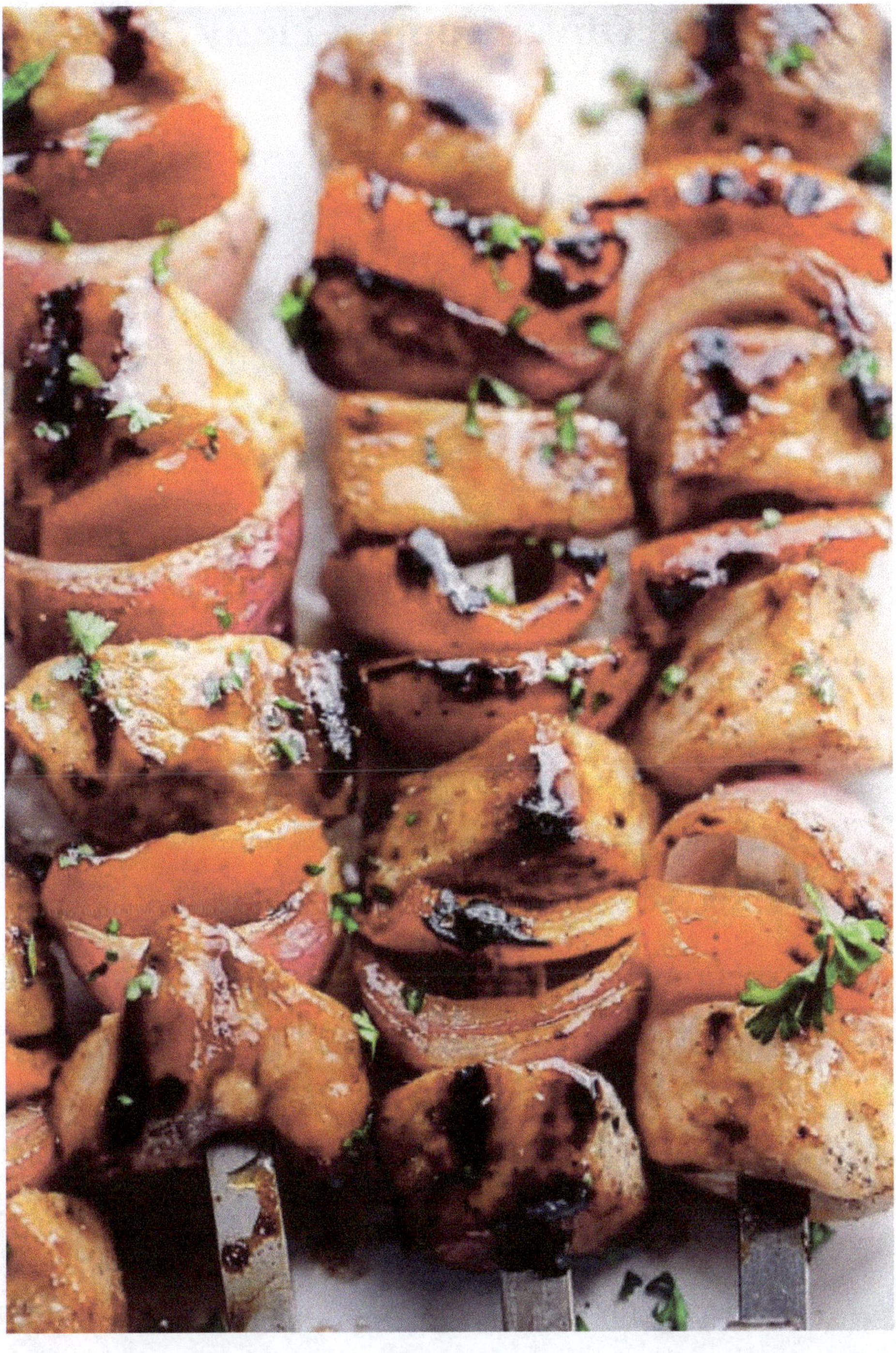

Capers 'n Olives Topped Flank Steak

Servings per Recipe: 4

Cooking Time: 45 minutes

Ingredients:

- 1 anchovy fillet, minced
- 1 clove of garlic, minced
- 1 cup pitted olives /250G
- 1 tablespoon capers, minced /15G
- 1/3 cup extra virgin olive oil /83ML
- 2 pounds flank steak, pounded /900G
- 2 tablespoons fresh oregano /30G
- 2 tablespoons garlic powder /30G
- 2 tablespoons onion powder /30G
- 2 tablespoons smoked paprika /30G
- Salt and pepper to taste

Instructions:

1) Preheat air fryer to 390° F or 199°C .
2) Place the grill pan in the mid-air fryer.
3) Season the steak with salt and pepper. Rub the oregano, paprika, onion powder, and garlic powder lavishly on the steak.
4) Place in the grill pan and cook for 45 minutes. Turnover the meat every 10 minutes to ensure even cooking.

5) Mix the olive oil, olives, capers, garlic, and anchovy fillets.
6) Serve the steak and dress using tapenade.

Nutrition information:

- Calories per serving: 553
- Carbs: 11.6g
- Protein: 51.5g
- Fat: 33.4g

Caraway, Sichuan 'n Cumin Lamb Kebabs

Servings per Recipe: 3

Cooking Time: 1 hour

Ingredients:

1 ½ pounds lamb shoulder, bones removed and cut into pieces /675G

1 tablespoon Sichuan peppercorns /15G

1 teaspoon sugar /5G

2 tablespoons cumin seeds, toasted /30G

2 teaspoons caraway seeds, toasted /10G

2 teaspoons crushed red pepper flakes /10G

Salt and pepper to taste

Instructions:

1) Place all ingredients in a bowl, add the meat and place in the fridge to marinate for a couple of hours.
2) Preheat mid-air fryer to 390° F or 199°C .
3) Place the grill pan in the air fryer.
4) Grill the meat for 15 minutes per batch.
5) Flip the meat every 8 minutes for even grilling.

Nutrition information:

- Calories per serving: 465
- Carbs:7.7g
- Protein: 22.8g
- Fat: 46.9g

Champagne-Vinegar Marinated Skirt Steak

Servings per Recipe: 2

Cooking Time: 40 minutes

Ingredients:

- ¼ cup Dijon mustard /32.5G
- 1 tablespoon rosemary leaves /15G
- 1-pound skirt steak, trimmed /450G
- 2 tablespoons champagne vinegar /30ML
- Salt and pepper to taste

Instructions:

1) Place all ingredients in a Ziploc bag and marinate in the fridge for a couple of hours.
2) Preheat air fryer to 390° F or 199°C .
3) Place the grill pan in the mid-air fryer.
4) Grill the skirt steak for 20 minutes per batch.
5) Flip the beef halfway through the cooking time.

Nutrition information:

- Calories per serving: 516
- Carbs: 4.2g
- Protein: 60.9g
- Fat: 28.4g

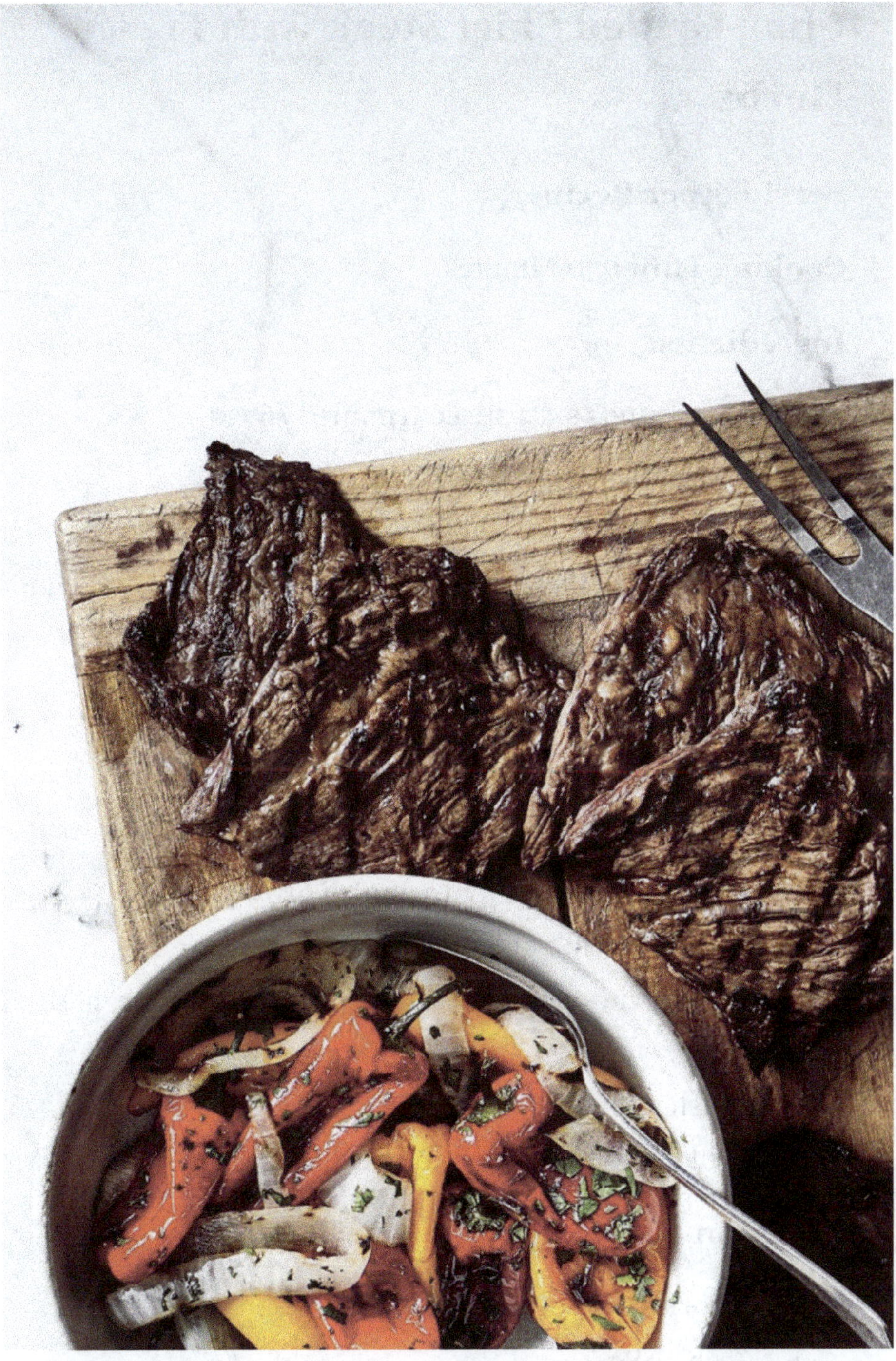

Char-Grilled Skirt Steak with Fresh Herbs

Servings per Recipe: 3

Cooking Time: 30 Minutes

Ingredients:

- 1 ½ pounds skirt steak, trimmed /675G
- 1 tablespoon lemon zest /15G
- 1 tablespoon olive oil /15G
- 2 cups fresh herbs like tarragon, sage, and mint, chopped /260G
- 4 cloves of garlic, minced
- Salt and pepper to taste

Instructions:

1) Preheat mid-air fryer to 390° F or 199°C .
2) Place the grill pan in the air fryer.
3) Season the steak with salt, pepper, lemon zest, herbs, and garlic.
4) Brush with oil.
5) Grill for 15 minutes and if needed cook in batches.

Nutrition information:

- Calories per serving: 478
- Carbs: 18g

- Protein: 25g
- Fat: 34g

Charred Onions 'n Steak Cube BBQ

Servings per Recipe: 3

Cooking Time: 40 minutes

Ingredients:

- 1 cup red onions, cut into wedges /130G
- 1 tablespoon dry mustard /15G
- 1 tablespoon organic olive oil /15ML
- 1-pound boneless beef sirloin, cut into cubes /450G
- Salt and pepper to taste

Instructions:

1) Preheat air fryer to 390° F or 199°C .
2) Place the grill pan in the air fryer.
3) Add all ingredients to the bowl and mix properly.
4) Place on the grill pan and cook for 40 minutes.
5) Shake halfway through the cooking time for even brownness.

Nutrition information:

- Calories per serving: 260
- Carbs: 5.2g
- Protein: 35.7g
- Fat: 10.7g

Cheddar Cheese ‘n Bacon Stuffed Pastry Pie

Servings per Recipe: 3

Cooking Time: 18 minutes

Ingredients:

- 1/2 cup bacon, cooked /65G
- 1/2 cup cheddar cheese, shredded /65G
- 1/2 cup sausage crumbles, cooked /65G
- 5 eggs
- one box puff pastry sheets

Instructions:

1) Scramble the eggs and cook.
2) Grease baking pan of air fryer lightly with cooking spray.
3) Evenly spread 50% of the puff sheets on the bottom of the pan.
4) Spread eggs, cooked sausage, crumbled bacon, and cheddar cheese.
5) top with remaining puff pastry and gently push down having a fork at the edges
6) Cover the surface of the baking pan with foil.
7) For 8 minutes, cook at 330° F or 166°C . Remove foil and continue cooking for an additional 5 minutes or until the tops of the puff pastry is golden brown.

8) Serve and enjoy.

Nutrition Information:

- Calories per Serving: 355
- Carbs: 9.4g
- Protein: 18.6g
- Fat: 26.9g

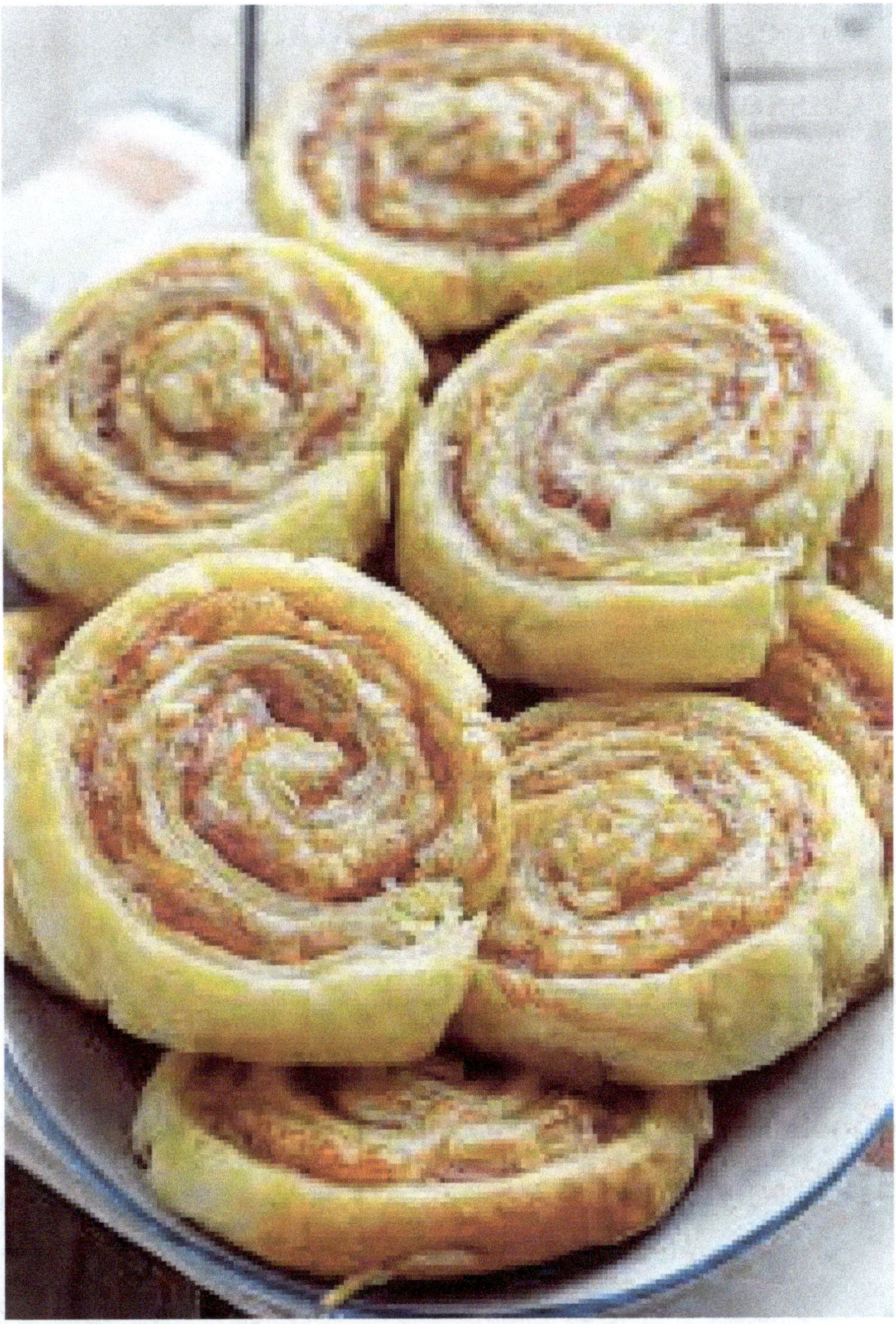

Cheesy Ground Beef 'n Mac Taco Casserole

Servings per Recipe: 5

Cooking Time: 25 minutes

Ingredients:

- 1-ounce shredded Cheddar cheese /30G
- 1-ounce shredded Monterey Jack cheese /30G
- 2 tablespoons chopped green onions /30G
- 1/2 (10.75 ounces) can condensed tomato soup /322.5ML
- 1/2-pound lean ground beef /225G
- 1/2 cup crushed tortilla chips /65G
- 1/4-pound macaroni, cooked as outlined by manufacturer's Instructions /112.5G
- 1/4 cup chopped onion /32.5G
- 1/4 cup sour cream (optional) /62.5ML
- 1/2 (1.25 ounce) package taco seasoning mix /37.5G
- 1/2 (14.5 ounces) can diced tomatoes /435G

Instructions:

1) Grease baking pan of air fryer lightly with cooking spray. Add onion and ground beef. For 10 minutes, cook on 360° F or 183°C . Stir and crush the ground beef halfway through cooking time.

2) Add taco seasoning, diced tomatoes, and tomato soup. Mix well. Mix in pasta.
3) Sprinkle crushed tortilla chips. Sprinkle cheese.
4) Cook for 15 minutes at 390° F or 199°C until tops are lightly browned and cheese is melted.
5) Serve and enjoy

Nutrition Information:

- Calories per Serving: 329
- Carbs: 28.2g
- Protein: 15.6g
- Fat: 17.0g

Cheesy Herbs Burger Patties

Servings per Recipe: 2

Cooking Time: 25 minutes

Ingredients:

- ¼ cup cheddar cheese /32.5G
- ½ teaspoon dried rosemary, crushed /2.5G
- 1-pound lean ground beef /450G
- 2 green onions, sliced thinly
- 2 tablespoons chopped parsley /30G
- 2 tablespoons ketchup /30ML
- 3 tablespoons Dijon mustard /45G
- 3 tablespoons dry breadcrumbs /45G
- Salt and pepper to taste

Instructions:

1) Combine all ingredients aside from the cheddar cheese in a mixing bowl. Mix well.
2) Mix properly using your hands to burger patties.
3) At the center of every patty, place a tablespoon of cheese and cover while using a meat mixture.
4) Preheat mid-air fryer to 390° F or 199°C .
5) Place the grill pan accessory and cook the patties for 25 minutes. Flip the patties halfway through the cooking time.

Nutrition information:

- Calories per serving: 358
- Carbs: 29g
- Protein: 29g
- Fat: 14g

Cheesy Potato Casserole the Amish Way

Servings per Recipe: 6

Cooking Time: 45 minutes

Ingredients:

- 2 cups frozen shredded hash brown potatoes, thawed /260G
- 5 medium eggs, lightly beaten
- 1 cup shredded Cheddar cheese /130G
- 1/2-pound sliced bacon, diced /225G
- 1/2 sweet onion, chopped
- 1/2 cup and two tablespoons shredded Swiss cheese /95G
- 3/4 cup small curd cottage cheese /88G

Instructions:

1) Oil baking pan of air fryer lightly with cooking spray.
2) For 10 minutes, cook at 330° F or 166°C of the onion and bacon. Eliminate excess fat.
3) Swiss cheese, some kinds of cheese, cheddar cheese, eggs, and potatoes. Pour into the pan of cooked bacon and mix well.
4) Cook for an additional 25 minutes.
5) Let it stay at home air fryer for one more 10 minutes.
6) Serve and enjoy

Nutrition Information:

- Calories per Serving: 341
- Carbs: 12.1g
- Protein: 21.7g
- Fat: 22.8g

Cheesy Sausage 'n Grits Bake From Down South

Servings per Recipe: 4

Cooking Time: 30 Minutes

Ingredients:

- 1/2 cup uncooked grits /65G
- 1/4-pound ground pork sausage /112.5G
- 1-1/2 cups water /375ML
- 2 tablespoons butter, divided /30G
- 2 tablespoons milk /30ML
- 3 eggs
- 3/4 cup shredded Cheddar cheese, divided /88G
- salt and pepper to taste

Instructions:

1) Place a large saucepan on heat, bring to a boil. Add in grits and simmer until liquid is absorbed around 5 minutes. Stir in ¼ cup cheese and 1 tbsp butter. Mix well until thoroughly combined.
2) Grease baking pan of air fryer lightly with cooking spray. Add pork sausage and then for 5 minutes, cook on 360° F or 183°C . Beat the sausage and remove excess fat.
3) Transfer grits into the pan containing sausage.

4) In a bowl, add milk and eggs, mix well, and pour into the pan. Mix well.
5) Add butter and sprinkle cheese. Season with pepper and salt.
6) Cook until tops are browned, around 20 minutes.
7) Serve and get.

Nutrition Information:

- Calories per Serving: 403
- Carbs: 16.8g
- Protein: 16.5g
- Fat: 29.9g

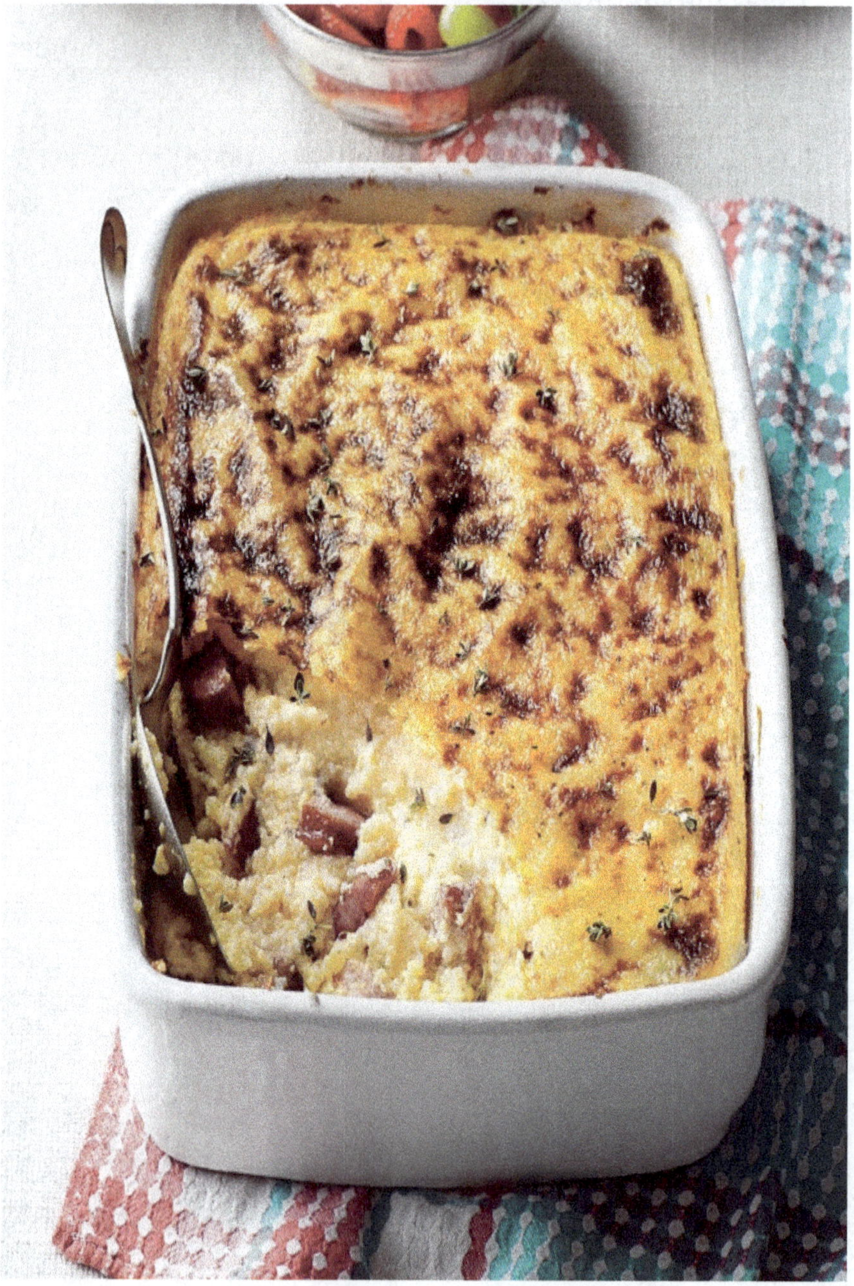

Chili-Espresso Marinated Steak

Servings per Recipe: 3

Cooking Time: 50 minutes

Ingredients:

- ½ teaspoon garlic powder /2.5G
- 1 ½ pounds beef flank steak /675G
- 1 teaspoon instant espresso powder /5G
- 2 tablespoons olive oil /30ML
- 2 teaspoons chili powder /10G
- Salt and pepper to taste

Instructions:

1) Preheat the air fryer to 390° F or 199°C .
2) Place the grill pan in the air fryer.
3) Mix the chili powder, salt, pepper, espresso powder, and garlic powder in a bowl.
4) Lavishly rub the seasoning on the steak and brush with oil.
5) Place on the grill pan and cook for 40 minutes.
6) Halfway from the cooking time, flip the beef to cook evenly.

Nutrition information:

- Calories per serving: 249
- Carbs: 4g

- Protein: 20g
- Fat: 17g

Chives on Bacon & Cheese Bake

Servings per Recipe: 6

Cooking Time: 50 minutes

Ingredients:

- 4 slices bread, crusts removed
- 1 cup egg substitute (for example Egg Beaters®) /250ML
- 1 tablespoon chopped fresh chives /15G
- 6 slices cooked bacon, crumbled
- 1 cup Cheddar cheese /130G
- 1 1/2 cups skim milk /375G

Instructions:

1) Cook bacon in a baking pan of air fryer for 10 minutes at 360° F or 183°C . Once done, remove excess fat then crush bacon.
2) Whisk eggs, stir in milk and chives.
3) In the same air fryer baking pan, evenly spread bread slices. Pour the egg mixture over it. Top with bacon. Cover the pan with foil and let it sit in the fridge for not less than 1 hour.
4) Preheat air fryer to 330° F or 166°C .
5) Cook while covered in foil for 20 Minutes. Remove foil and sprinkle cheese. Continue cooking uncovered for an additional 15 minutes.

6) Serve and enjoy

Nutrition Information:

- Calories per Serving: 207
- Carbs: 12.1g
- Protein: 15.3g
- Fat: 10.8g

Cilantro-Mint Pork BBQ Thai Style

Servings per Recipe: 3

Cooking Time: 15 minutes

Ingredients:

- 1 minced hot chile
- 1 minced shallot
- 1-pound ground pork /450G
- 2 tablespoons fish sauce /30ML
- 2 tablespoons lime juice /30ML
- 3 tablespoons basil /45G
- 3 tablespoons chopped mint /45G
- 3 tablespoons cilantro /45G

Instructions:

1) Place all ingredients in a shallow dish, using your hands mix properly and make 1-inch balls.
2) Skewer the balls and place them on the skewer rack in the air fryer.
3) For 15 minutes, cook on 360° F or 183°C . Halfway through cooking time, turnover skewers. If needed, cook in batches.
4) Serve and enjoy

Nutrition Information:

- Calories per Serving: 455
- Carbs: 2.5g
- Protein: 40.2g
- Fat: 31.5g

Coriander Lamb with Pesto 'n Mint Dip

Servings per Recipe: 4

Cooking Time: 16 minutes

Ingredients:

- 1 1/2 teaspoons coriander seeds, ground in a spice mill or perhaps mortar with pestle /7.5G
- 1 large red bell pepper, cut into 1-inch squares
- 1 small red onion, cut into 1-inch squares
- 1 tablespoon extra-virgin extra virgin olive oil plus additional for brushing /15ML
- 1 teaspoon coarse kosher salt /5G
- 1-pound trimmed lamb meat, cut into 1 1/4-inch cube /450G
- 4 large garlic cloves, minced

Mint-Pesto Dip Ingredients:

- 1 cup (packed) fresh mint leaves /130G
- 2 tablespoons pine nuts /30G
- 2 tablespoons freshly grated Parmesan cheese /30G
- 1 tablespoon fresh lemon juice /15ML
- 1 medium garlic herb, peeled
- 1/2 cup (packed) fresh cilantro leaves /65G
- 1/2 teaspoon coarse kosher salt /2.5G
- 1/2 cup (or even more) extra-virgin olive oil /65ML

Instructions:

1) In a blender, puree all Mint-Pesto dip Ingredients until smooth and creamy. Transfer to a bowl and set aside.
2) Mix coriander, salt, garlic, and oil in a large bowl. Add lamb, mix well to coat. Place in a fridge and allow to marinate for no less than 1 hour.
3) Thread lamb, bell pepper, and onion alternately in a skewer. Repeat until all ingredients are used. Place in skewer rack in the air fryer.
4) For 8 minutes, cook at 390° F or 199°C . Halfway through cooking time, turnover.
5) Serve and dress with sauce.

Nutrition Information:

- Calories per Serving: 307
- Carbs: 6.3g
- Protein: 21.1g
- Fat: 21.9

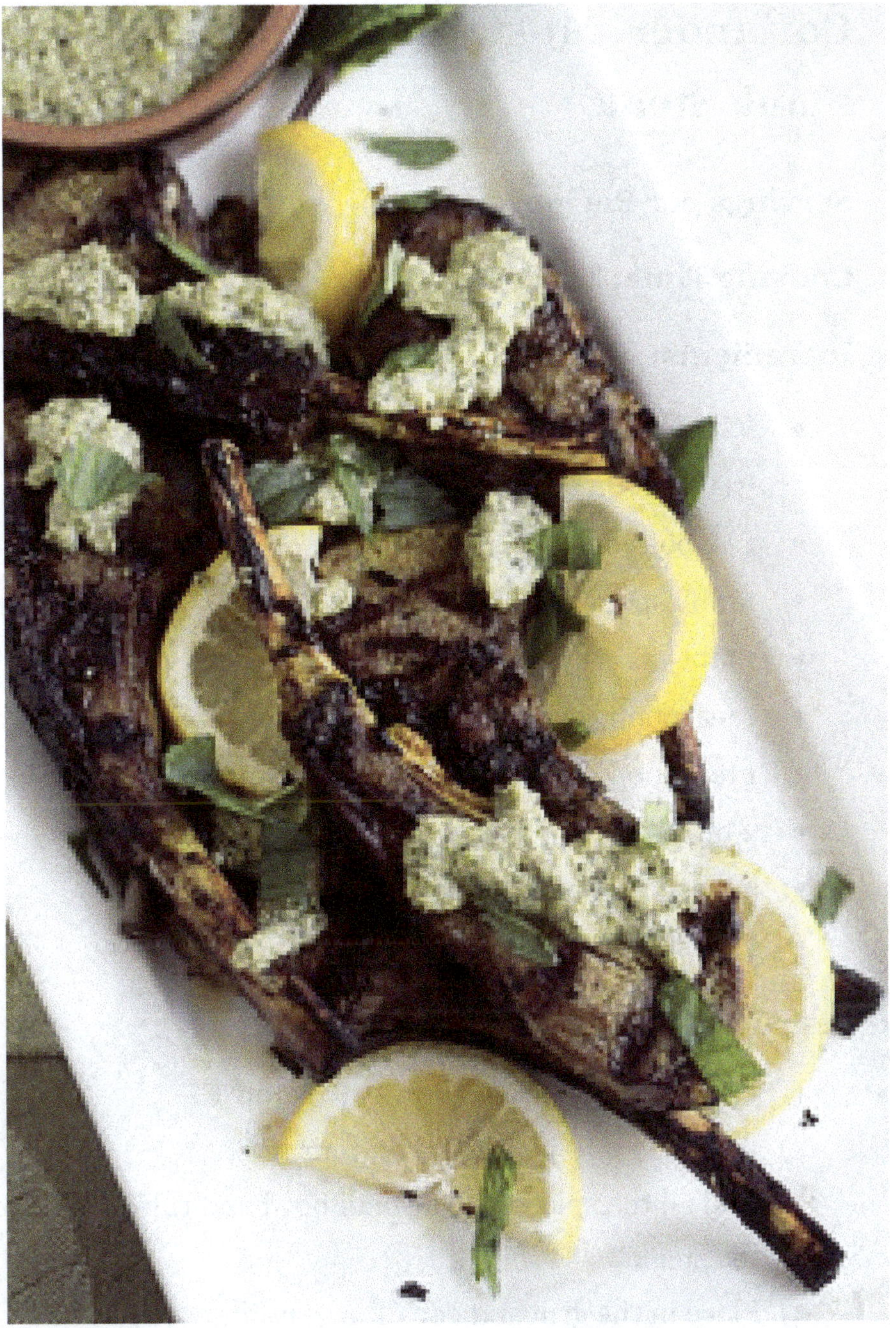

Coriander, Mustard 'n Cumin Rubbed Flank Steak

Servings per Recipe: 3

Cooking Time: 45 minutes

Ingredients:

- ½ teaspoon coriander /2.5G
- ½ teaspoon ground cumin /2.5G
- 1 ½ pounds flank steak /675G
- 1 tablespoon chili powder /15G
- 1 tablespoon paprika /15G
- 1 teaspoon garlic powder /5G
- 1 teaspoon mustard powder /5G
- 2 tablespoons sugar /30G
- 2 teaspoons black pepper /10G
- 2 teaspoons salt /10G

Instructions:

1) Preheat the air fryer to 390° F or 199°C .
2) Place the grill pan in the mid-air fryer.
3) Add all the spices into a small bowl and rub lavishly on the steak.
4) Place in the grill and cook for 15 minutes per batch.
5) Turn over the meat every 8 minutes for even grilling.

Nutrition information:

- Calories per serving: 330
- Carbs: 10.2g
- Protein:50 g
- Fat:12.1 g

Cornbread, Ham 'n Eggs Frittata

Servings per Recipe: 3

Cooking Time: 45 minutes

Ingredients:

- 1 stalk celery, diced
- 1/2 (14.5 ounces) can chicken broth /435ML
- 1/2 (14-ounce) package seasoned cornbread stuffing mix /420G
- 1/2 cup chopped onion /65G
- 1/4 cup butter /32.5G
- 1/4 cup water /62.5G
- 1/4 teaspoon paprika, for garnish /2.5G
- 2 cups diced cooked ham /260G
- 3 eggs
- 3/4 cup shredded Cheddar cheese /88G

Instructions:

1) Oil the baking pan of the air fryer lightly with cooking spray. Add celery and onions.
2) For 5 minutes, cook at 360° F or 183°C . Stir in ham. Cook for an additional 5 minutes.
3) Stir in butter, water, and chicken broth. Mix well and keep cooking for an additional 5 minutes.

4) Throw in the stuffing mix and mix well to coat. Cover pan with foil.
5) Cook for 15 minutes.
6) Remove foil to make 3 indentations inside the stuffing to keep an egg. Break an egg in each hole.
7) Cook uncovered for the next 10 minutes or until egg is cooked to desired doneness.
8) Sprinkle with cheese and paprika. Let it cook in the air fryer for an additional 5 minutes.
9) Serve and enjoy.

Nutrition Information:

- Calories per Serving: 847
- Carbs: 54.4g
- Protein: 37.5g
- Fat: 53.2g

Country Style Sausage & Hash Browns

Servings per Recipe: 4

Cooking Time: 45 minutes

Ingredients:

- 1 cup shredded Cheddar cheese /130G
- 1 stalk green onion, chopped
- 1/2 (2.64-ounce) package country gravy mix /79ML
- 1/2 cup milk /125ML
- 3 eggs, lightly beaten
- 8-ounce bulk breakfast sausage /240G
- 8-ounce package hash brown potatoes /240G
- A dash of paprika as well as to taste (optional)

Instructions:

1) Grease the baking pan of the air fryer lightly with cooking spray.
2) For 10 minutes, grind and cook sausage at 360° F or 183°C . Halfway through cooking time, open the air fryer and continue grinding sausage.
3) When cooked, drain excess oil.
4) Stir in green onions and evenly spread ground sausage. Spread hash brown potatoes and sprinkle cheese evenly.
5) Whisk gravy, milk, and eggs in a bowl until smooth. Pour over cheese mixture. Sprinkle top with paprika.

6) Cover the pan with foil.
7) Cook for 20 minutes, remove foil and cook for another 10 Minutes.
8) Let it sit for 5 minutes.
9) Serve and enjoy

Nutrition Information:

- Calories per Serving: 406
- Carbs: 13.3g
- Protein: 21.7g
- Fat: 29.5g

Crispy Fried Pork Chops the Southern Way

Servings per Recipe: 4

Cooking Time: 25 minutes

Ingredients:

- ½ cup all-purpose flour /65G
- ½ cup low-fat buttermilk /125ML
- ½ teaspoon black pepper /2.5G
- 1 ½ teaspoon Tabasco sauce /7.5ML
- 1 teaspoon paprika /5G
- **4 bone-in pork chops**

Instructions:

1) Place the buttermilk and hot sauce in a Ziploc bag and add the pork chops. Allow to marinate for about one hour in the fridge.
2) Add the flour, paprika, and black pepper to a bowl and mix well.
3) Remove pork from the Ziploc bag and dredge in the flour mixture.
4) Preheat the air fryer to 390° F or 199°C .
5) Spray the pork chops with oil.
6) Place in an air fryer basket and cook for 25 minutes.

Nutrition information:

- Calories per serving: 427
- Carbs:12.6 g
- Protein: 46.4g
- Fat: 21.2g

Crispy Roast Garlic-Salt Pork

Servings per Recipe: 4

Cooking Time: 45 minutes

Ingredients:

- 1 teaspoon Chinese five-spice powder /5G
- 1 teaspoon white pepper /5G
- 2 pounds pork belly /900G
- 2 teaspoons garlic salt /10G

Instructions:

1) Preheat the air fryer to 390° F or 199°C .
2) To make the dry rub, mix all the spices in a bowl.
3) Remove the skin layer from the pork belly and season the entire pork with all the spice rub.
4) Place in the mid-air fryer basket and cook for 40 to 45 minutes before the skin is crispy.
5) Chop into bits before serving.

Nutrition information:

- Calories per serving: 785
- Carbs: 0.7g
- Protein: 14.2g
- Fat: 80.7g

Cumin 'n Chili Rubbed Steak Fajitas

Servings per Recipe: 2

Cooking Time: 25 minutes

Ingredients:

- ¼ teaspoon chili powder /1.25G
- ¼ teaspoon oregano /1.25G
- ½ cup cotija cheese /65G
- ½ medium red onion, chopped
- ½ teaspoon ground cumin /2.5G
- 1 small bell pepper
- 1-pound sliced beef, cut into strips /450G
- 2 chopped serrano peppers
- 2 tablespoons extra virgin olive oil /30ML
- Corn tortillas
- Salt and pepper to taste

Instructions:

1) Preheat air fryer to 390° F or 199°C .
2) Place the grill pan in the air fryer.
3) Add the beef to a mixing bowl and season with salt, pepper, oregano, ground cumin, chili powder, and extra virgin olive oil.
4) Place in the grill pan and cook for 25 minutes.

5) Halfway through the cooking time, stir the meat to cook evenly.
6) Once cooked, serve the beef with corn tortillas, cheese, and Serrano peppers.

Nutrition information:

- Calories per serving: 599
- Carbs: 16.8g
- Protein: 54.9g
- Fat: 34.7

Cumin-Paprika Rubbed Beef Brisket

Serves: 12

Cooking Time: a couple of hours

Ingredients:

- ¼ teaspoon cayenne pepper /1.25G
- 1 ½ tablespoons paprika /22.5G
- 1 teaspoon garlic powder /5G
- 1 teaspoon ground cumin /5G
- 1 teaspoon onion powder /5G
- 2 teaspoons dry mustard /10G
- 2 teaspoons ground black pepper /10G
- 2 teaspoons salt /10G
- 5 pounds brisket roast /2250G
- 5 tablespoons extra virgin olive oil /75ML

Instructions:

1) Place all ingredients inside a Ziploc bag and marinate inside the fridge for at least a couple of hours.
2) Preheat the air fryer for 5 minutes.
3) Place the meat in a baking dish that may easily fit into a mid-air fryer.
4) Place in the air fryer and cook for 120 minutes at 350° F or 177°C .

Nutrition information:

- Calories per serving: 269
- Carbohydrates: 2.8g
- Protein: 35.6g
- Fat: 12.8g

Cumin-Sichuan Lamb BBQ with Dip

Servings per Recipe: 4

Cooking Time: 25 minutes

BBQ Ingredients:

- 1 1/4 pounds boneless lamb shoulder, cut into 1-inch pieces /562.5G
- 1 tablespoon Sichuan peppercorns or 1 teaspoon black peppercorns /15G
- 1 teaspoon sugar /5G
- 2 tablespoons cumin seeds /30G
- 2 teaspoons caraway seeds /10G
- 2 teaspoons crushed red pepper flakes /10G
- Finely grated lemon zest (for serving)
- Kosher salt, freshly cracked pepper

For the Garlic Yogurt Dip:

- 1 garlic oil, grated
- 1 tablespoon fresh freshly squeezed lemon juice /15ML
- 1 cup plain Greek yogurt /250ML
- Kosher salt, freshly ground pepper
- 1/2 teaspoon finely grated lemon zest /2.5G

Instructions:

1) Process cumin seeds, peppercorns, caraway seeds, pepper flakes, and sugar until smooth in a processor.
2) Thread lamb pieces into skewers. Season with salt. Rub paste throughout meat pieces.
3) Place on skewer rack.
4) Cook for 5 minutes at 390° F or 199°C or desired doneness.
5) Meanwhile, in a medium bowl whisk well dip Ingredients and set aside.
6) Serve and enjoy with dip.

Nutrition Information:

- Calories per Serving: 265
- Carbs: 7.6g
- Protein: 34.3g
- Fat: 10.8g

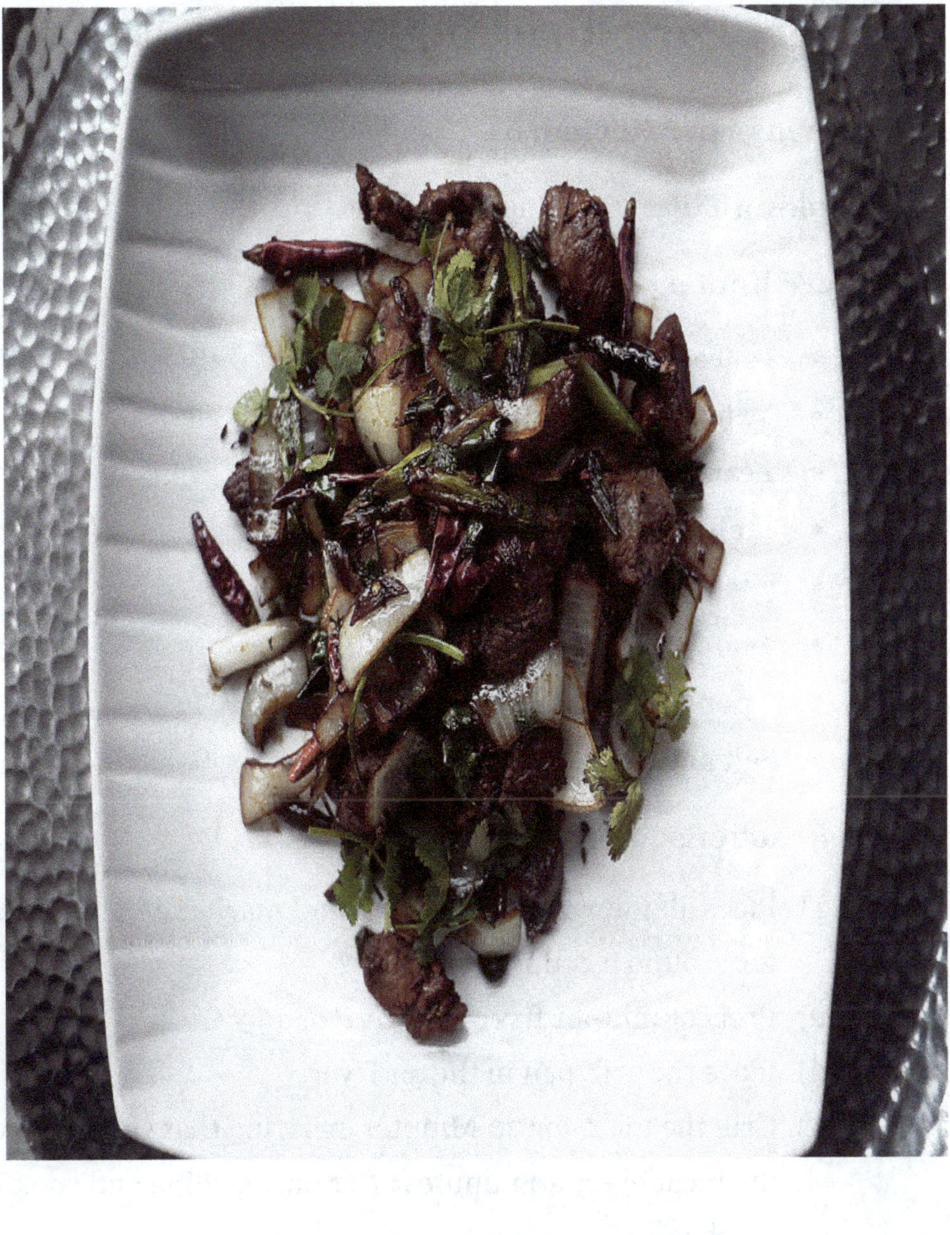

Curry Pork Roast in Coconut Sauce

Servings per Recipe: 6

Cooking Time: 60 Minutes

Ingredients:

- ½ teaspoon curry powder /2.5G
- ½ teaspoon ground turmeric powder /2.5G
- 1 can of unsweetened coconut milk
- 1 tablespoons sugar /15G
- 2 tablespoons fish sauce /30ML
- 2 tablespoons soy sauce /30ML
- 3 pounds pork shoulder /1350G
- Salt and pepper to taste

Instructions:

1) Place all ingredients in a bowl and marinate in the fridge for around a couple of hours.
2) Preheat mid-air fryer to 390° F or 199°C .
3) Place the grill pan in the air fryer.
4) Grill the meat for 20 Minutes ensuring that you turn over the meat every 10 minutes after only grilling and cook in batches.
5) Meanwhile, pour the marinade in a saucepan and simmer for 10 minutes before the sauce thickens.
6) Baste the pork using the sauce before serving.

Nutrition information:

- Calories per serving: 688
- Carbs: 38g
- Protein: 17g
- Fat: 52g

Eastern Chunky Shish Kebabs

Servings per Recipe: 4

Cooking Time: 20 minutes

Ingredients:

- 1 tablespoon prepared mustard /15G
- 1 tablespoon Worcestershire sauce /15ML
- 1 clove garlic, minced
- 1 teaspoon coarsely cracked black pepper /5G
- 16 mushroom caps
- 2 green sweet peppers, cut into chunks
- 1 red bell pepper, cut into chunks
- 1 large onion, cut into large squares
- 1/2 cup soy sauce /125ML
- 1 1/2 teaspoons salt /7.5G
- 1 1/2 pounds lean beef, cut into 1-inch cubes /675G
- 1/3 cup vegetable oil /188ML
- 1/4 cup lemon juice /62.5G

Instructions:

1) Mix salt, pepper, garlic, Worcestershire, mustard, lemon juice, soy sauce, and oil properly in a bowl. Add beef and mix well to coat. Remove excess air and seal. Marinate for 8 hours. Add mushroom and marinate for an additional 8 hours.

2) Thread mushrooms, bell peppers, onion, and meat in skewers.
3) Pour marinade in a saucepan and thicken for 10 minutes and transfer to some bowl for basting.
4) Place skewers on the skewer rack in the air fryer. If needed, cook in batches.
5) For 10, cook on 390° F or 199°C . Halfway through cooking time, baste and turnover skewers.
6) Serve and enjoy

Nutrition Information:

- Calories per Serving: 426
- Carbs: 15.8g
- Protein: 26.2g
- Fat: 28.6g

Easy & The Traditional Beef Roast Recipe

Serves: 12

Cooking Time: 120 minutes

Ingredients:

- 1 cup organic beef broth /250ML
- 3 pounds beef round roast /1350G
- 4 tablespoons essential olive oil /60ML
- Salt and pepper to taste

Instructions:

1) Put all ingredients in a Ziploc bag, allow to marinate in the fridge for 2 hours.
2) Preheat mid-air fryer for 5 minutes.
3) Transfer all ingredients to a baking dish that may fit in the air fryer.
4) Place in the air fryer and cook for 2 hours for 400° F or 205°C .

Nutrition information:

- Calories per serving: 284
- Carbohydrates:0.4 g
- Protein: 23.7g
- Fat: 20.8g

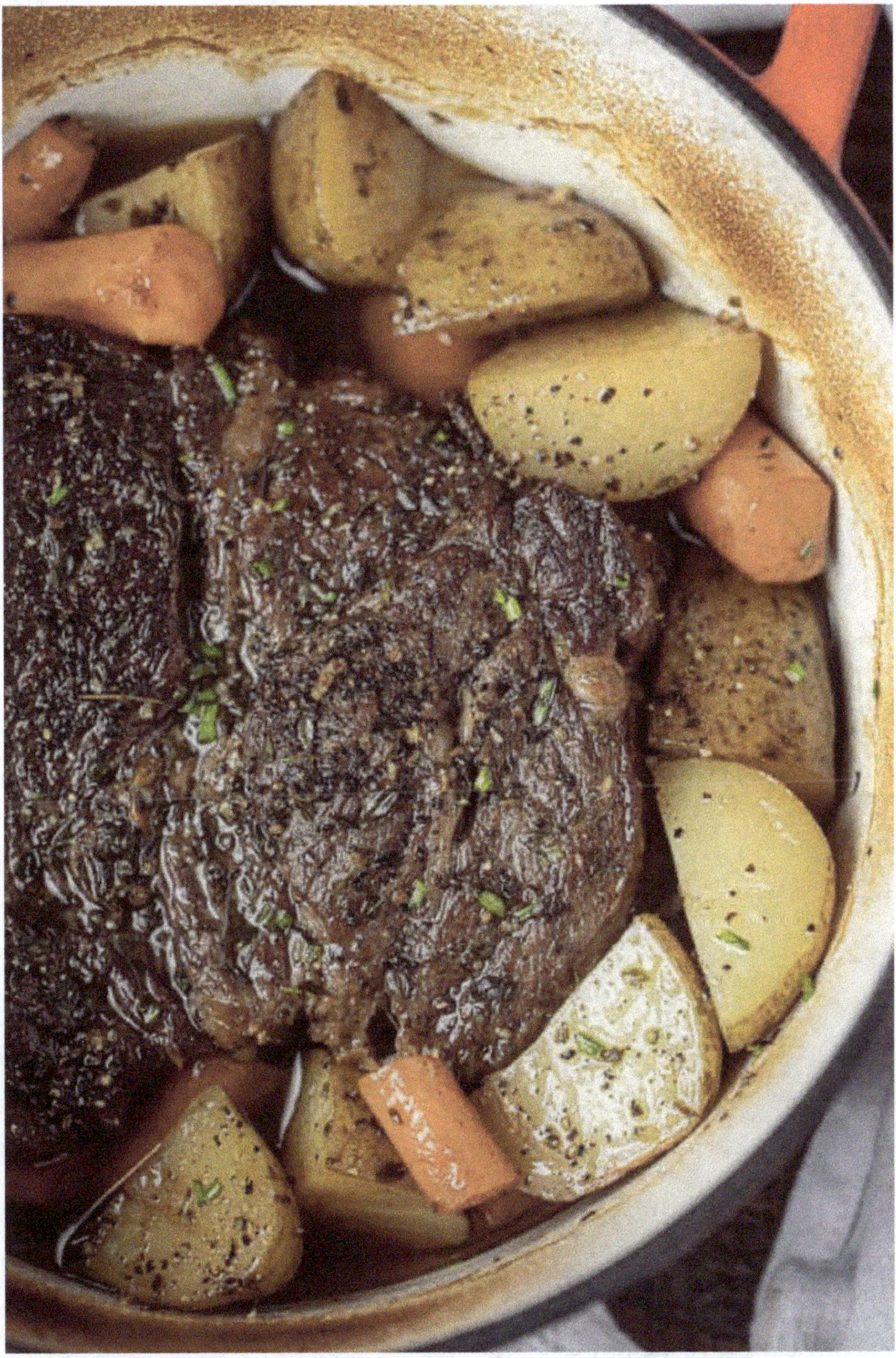

Easy Corn Dog Bites

Servings per Recipe: 2

Cooking Time: 10

Ingredients:

- ½ cup all-purpose flour /65G
- 1 ½ cup crushed cornflakes /195G
- 2 large beef sausages, cut by 50 per cent crosswise
- 2 large eggs, beaten
- Salt and pepper to taste

Instructions

1) Preheat the air fryer to 330° F or 166°C .
2) Skewer the sausages with a mental skewer that came with the double layer rack accessory.
3) In a mixing bowl, combine the flour and eggs to create a batter. Season with salt and pepper to taste. Add water if too dry.
4) Dip the skewered sausages in the batter and dredge in cornflakes.
5) Place in the double layer rack and cook for 10 minutes.

Nutrition information:

- Calories per serving: 79

- Carbs:8 g
- Protein: 5g
- Fat: 3g

Egg Noodles, Ground Beef & Tomato Sauce Bake

Servings per Recipe: 3

Cooking Time: 45 minutes

Ingredients:

- 1 (15 ounces) can tomato sauce /450ML
- 4-ounce egg noodles, cooked according to manufacturer's directions /120G
- 1/2-pound ground beef /225G
- 1/2 teaspoon white sugar /2.5G
- 1/2 teaspoon salt /2.5G
- 1/2 teaspoon garlic salt /2.5G
- 1/2 cup sour cream /125ML
- 1/2 large white onion, diced
- 1/4 cup shredded sharp Cheddar cheese, or higher to taste /32.5G
- 1.5-ounce cream cheese /45G

Instructions:

1) Grease the baking pan of the air fryer lightly with cooking spray. Add ground beef, for 10 minutes cook on 360° F or 183°C . Halfway through cooking time crush beef.
2) When done cooking, remove excess fat.

3) Stir in tomato sauce, garlic salt, salt, and sugar. Mix well and cook for the next 15 minutes. Transfer to a bowl.
4) Whisk onion, cream cheese, and sour cream properly in a bowl.
5) Place half of the egg noodles on the bottom of the air fryer baking pan. Top with 50 % of the sour cream mixture, then half the tomato sauce mixture. Repeat layering. And then top of with cheese.
6) Cover the pan with foil.
7) Cook for the next 15 minutes. Uncover and cook for the next 5 minutes.
8) Serve and enjoy

Nutrition Information:

- Calories per Serving: 524
- Carbs: 39.4g
- Protein: 24.5g
- Fat: 29.8g

Eggs 'n Bacon on Biscuit Brekky

Servings per Recipe: 4

Cooking Time: 28 minutes

Ingredients:

- ¼ cup milk /62.5ML
- ½ of 16-ounces refrigerated breakfast biscuits /240G
- 1 cup shredded extra-sharp cheddar cheese /130G
- 4 scallions, chopped
- 5 eggs
- 8 slices cooked center cut bacon

Instructions:

1) Set the pan over heat and cook for 8 minutes at 360° F or 183°C or until crisped. Remove bacon and discard excess fat.
2) Evenly spread biscuits on the bottom of the basket. For 5 minutes, cook at 360° F or 183°C .
3) Meanwhile, whisk eggs, milk, and scallions in a bowl.
4) Remove basket, evenly layer bacon ahead of biscuit, sprinkle cheese on top, and pour eggs.
5) Cook for 15 minutes or until eggs are set.
6) Serve and enjoy

Nutrition Information:

- Calories per Serving: 241
- Carbs: 4.3g
- Protein: 22.6g
- Fat: 23.7g

Fat Burger Bombs

Serves: 6

Cooking Time: 20 Minutes

Ingredients:

- ½ pound ground beef /225G
- 1 cup almond flour /130G
- 12 slices uncured bacon, chopped
- 2 eggs, beaten
- 3 tablespoons olive oil /45ML
- Salt and pepper to taste

Instructions:

1) In a mixing bowl, combine all ingredients aside from the olive oil.
2) Use your hands to make small balls with the mixture. Place in the baking sheet and allow to marinate and put in the fridge for about 2 hours.
3) Preheat mid-air fryer for 5 minutes.
4) Brush the meatballs with olive oil on all sides.
5) Place in the air fryer basket.
6) Cook for 20 minutes at 350° F or 177°C .
7) Halfway through the cooking time, shake the fryer basket for a more even cooking.

Nutrition information:

- Calories per serving: 412
- Carbohydrates: 1.5g
- Protein: 19.2g
- Fat: 36.6g

Flatiron Steak Grill on Parsley Salad

Servings per Recipe: 4

Cooking Time: 45 minutes

Ingredients:

- ½ cup mozzarella, grated /65G
- 1 ½ pounds flatiron steak /675G
- 1 tablespoon fresh freshly squeezed lemon juice /15ML
- 2 cups parsley leaves /260G
- 3 tablespoons olive oil /45ML
- Salt and pepper to taste

Instructions:

1) Preheat the air fryer to 390° F or 199°C .
2) Place the grill pan in the mid-air fryer.
3) Mix the steak, oil, salt and pepper.
4) Grill for 15 minutes per batch making sure to turn over the meat halfway through the cooking time.
5) Meanwhile, combine the parsley leaves, parmesan cheese and fresh lemon juice to make the salad. Season with salt and pepper.

Nutrition information:

- Calories per serving: 595
- Carbs: 4.9g

- Protein: 47g
- Fat: 43g

Fried Pork with Sweet and Sour Glaze

Servings per Recipe: 4

Cooking Time: 30 Minutes

Ingredients:

- ¼ cup rice wine vinegar /62.5ML
- ¼ teaspoon Chinese five-spice powder /1.25G
- 1 cup potato starch /250G
- 1 green onion, chopped
- 2 large eggs, beaten
- 2 pounds pork chops cut into chunks /900G
- 2 tablespoons cornstarch + 3 tablespoons water /30G+ 45ML
- 5 tablespoons brown sugar /75G
- Salt and pepper to taste

Instructions:

1) Preheat mid-air fryer to 390° F or 199°C .
2) Season pork chops with salt and pepper to taste.
3) Dip the pork chops in egg. Set aside.
4) In a bowl, combine the potato starch and Chinese five-spice powder.
5) Dredge the pork chops in the flour mixture.
6) Place in the double layer rack and cook for a half-hour.

7) Meanwhile, put the vinegar and brown sugar in the saucepan. Season with salt and pepper to taste. Stir in the cornstarch slurry and allow to simmer for 10 minutes.
8) Serve the pork chops while using sauce and garnish with green onions.

Nutrition information:

- Calories per serving: 420
- Carbs: 9.1g
- Protein: 69.2g
- Fat: 11.8g

Garlic Lemon-Wine on Lamb Steak

Servings per Recipe: 4

Cooking Time: an hour and 30 Minutes

Ingredients:

- ¼ cup extra virgin essential olive oil /62.5ML
- ½ cup dry white wine /65G
- 1 tablespoon brown sugar /15G
- 2 pounds lamb steak, pounded /900G
- 2 tablespoons lemon juice /30ML
- 3 tablespoons ancho chili powder /45G
- 8 cloves of garlic, minced
- Salt and pepper to taste

Instructions:

1) Place all ingredients in a bowl and allow the meat to marinate by placing it in a fridge for a couple of hours.
2) Preheat mid-air fryer to 390° F or 199°C .
3) Place the grill pan in the air fryer.
4) Grill the meat for 20 minutes per batch.
5) Meanwhile, pour the marinade in a saucepan and allow to simmer for 10 minutes.

Nutrition information:

- Calories per serving: 500

- Carbs: 8g
- Protein: 38g
- Fat: 35g

Garlic-Cumin 'n Orange Juice Marinated Steak

Servings per Recipe: 4

Cooking Time: one hour

Ingredients:

- ¼ cup orange juice /62.5ML
- 1 teaspoon ground cumin /5G
- 2 pounds skirt steak, trimmed from body fat /900G
- 2 tablespoons lime juice /30ML
- 2 tablespoons organic olive oil /30ML
- 4 cloves of garlic, minced
- Salt and pepper to taste

Instructions:

1) Place all ingredients in a mixing bowl and allow to marinate by placing the bowl in a fridge for a couple of hours.
2) Preheat air fryer to 390° F or 199°C .
3) Place the grill pan in the mid-air fryer.
4) Grill for 15 minutes per batch and flip the beef every 8 minutes to ensure even grilling.
5) Meanwhile, pour the marinade on a saucepan and allow to simmer for 10 minutes or before the sauce thickens.
6) Slice the beef and pour in the sauce.

Nutrition information:

- Calories per serving: 568
- Carbs: 4.7g
- Protein: 59.1g
- Fat: 34.7g

Garlicky Buttered Chops

Servings per Recipe: 4

Cooking Time: 30 Minutes

Ingredients:

- 1 tablespoon butter, melted /15ML
- 2 teaspoons chopped parsley /10G
- 2 teaspoons grated garlic /10G
- 4 pork chops
- Salt and pepper to taste

Instructions:

1) Preheat mid-air fryer to 330° F or 166°C .
2) Place the grill pan in the air fryer.
3) Use the remaining ingredients to season the pork chops while.
4) Place on the grill pan and cook for 30 minutes.
5) Flip the pork chops every 15 minutes.

Nutrition information:

- Calories per serving: 352
- Carbs: 1.6g
- Protein: 40.7g
- Fat: 20.3g

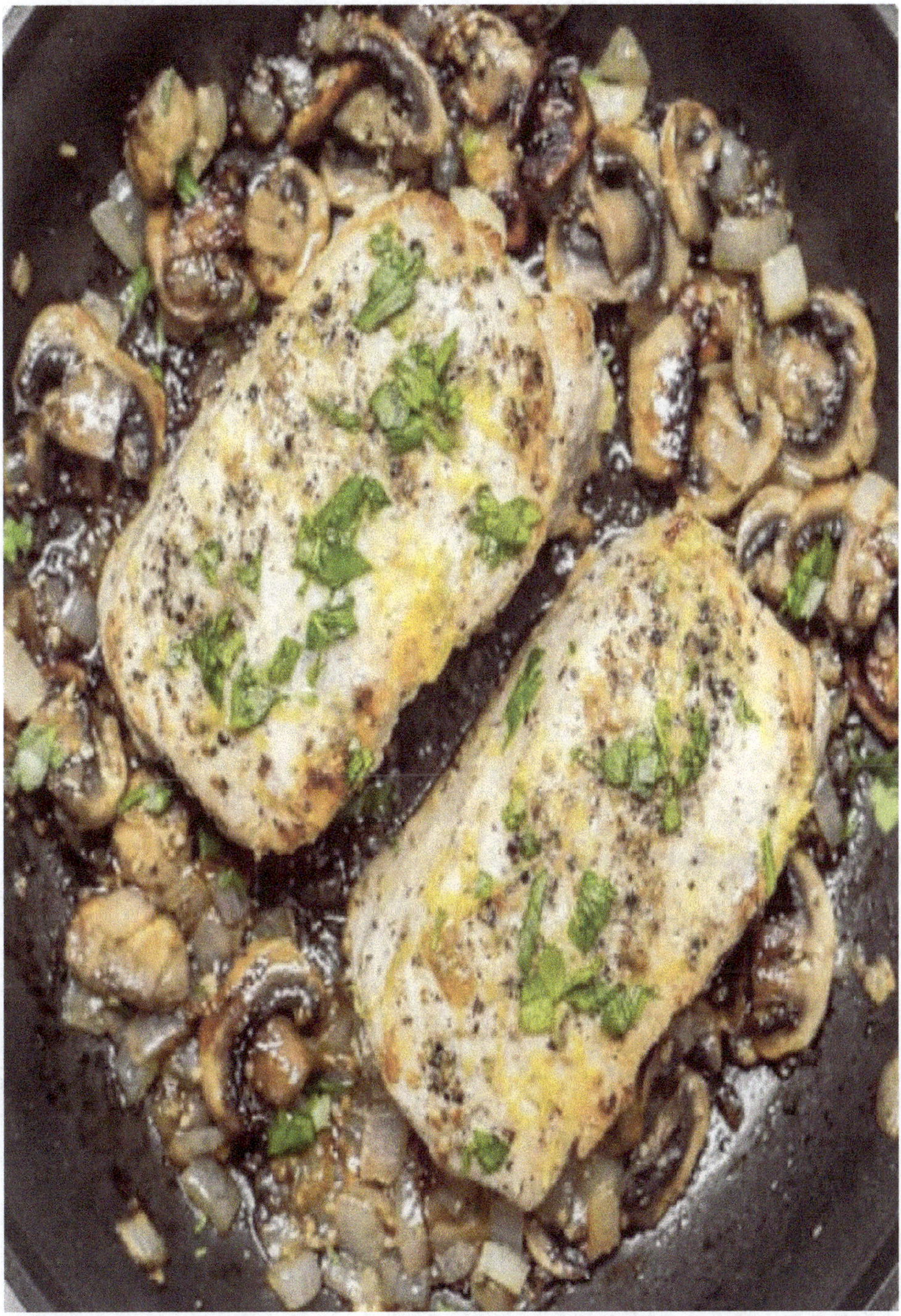

Garlic-Mustard Rubbed Roast Beef

Serves: 12

Cooking Time: 120 minutes

Ingredients:

- ¼ cup Dijon mustard /32.5G
- ¼ cup freshly parsley, chopped /32.5G
- ¼ cup unsalted butter /32.5G
- 2 cups almond flour /260G
- 2 tablespoons olive oil /30ML
- 3 ½ cups beef broth /875ML
- 3 pounds boneless beef eye round roast /1350G
- 4 cloves of garlic, chopped
- Salt and pepper to taste

Instructions:

1) Add the garlic, almond flour, parsley, salt and pepper to a bowl.
2) Place a pan on heat, add butter and essential olive oil, place the beef in the pan allow it to brown on every side.
3) Rub the almond flour mixture around the beef.
4) Brush with Dijon mustard.
5) Place the crusted beef in a baking dish.
6) Pour the beef broth slowly.
7) Place the baking dish in the air fryer.

8) Cook for 120 minutes at 400° F or 205°C .
9) Baste the beef with the sauce every 30 minutes.

Nutrition information:

- Calories per serving: 310
- Carbohydrates: 7.2g
- Protein: 24.6g
- Fat: 20.30g

Garlic-Rosemary Lamb BBQ

Servings per Recipe: 2

Cooking Time: 12 minutes

Ingredients:

- 1-lb cubed lamb leg /450G
- juice of merely one lemon
- fresh rosemary
- 3 smashed garlic cloves
- salt and pepper
- 1/2 cup organic olive oil /125ML

Instructions:

1) Mix all the ingredients in a shallow bowl and marinate for 3 hours.
2) Skewer the lamb pieces. Place on skewer rack in the air fryer.
3) For 12 minutes, cook on 390° F or 199°C . Turnover skewers every 6 minutes. If need be, cook in batches.
4) Serve and enjoy

Nutrition Information:

- Calories per Serving: 560
- Carbs: 5.4g
- Protein: 46.5g
- Fat: 39.1g

Garlic-Rosemary Rubbed Beef Rib Roast

Serves: 14

Cooking Time: a couple of hours

Ingredients:

- 1 cup dried porcini mushrooms /130G
- 1 medium shallot, chopped
- 2 cloves of garlic, minced
- 2 cups water /500ML
- 3 tablespoons unsalted pepper /45G
- 3 tablespoons vegetable oil /45ML
- 4 sprigs of thyme
- 6 ribs, beef rib roast
- Salt and pepper to taste

Instructions:

1) Preheat the air fryer for 5 minutes.
2) Place all ingredients in the baking dish that can easily fit in the air fryer.
3) Place the dish in the air fryer and cook for a couple of hours at 325° F or 163°C .

Nutrition information:

- Calories per serving: 320
- Carbohydrates: 0.9g

- Protein: 32.4g
- Fat: 20.7g

Ginger Soy Beef Recipe in the Orient

Servings per Recipe: 3

Cooking Time: 5 minutes

Ingredients:

- 2 tablespoons soy sauce /30ML
- 1 green onions, chopped
- 1 clove garlic, minced
- 1 tablespoon and 1-1/2 teaspoons hoisin sauce /22.5ML
- 1 tablespoon and 1-1/2 teaspoons sherry /22.5ML
- ·1/2 teaspoon barbeque sauce /2.5ML
- 1-1/2 teaspoons minced fresh ginger root /7.5G
- 3/4-pound flank steak, thinly sliced /337.5G

Instructions:

1) Add the ginger, garlic, green onions, barbecue sauce, soy sauce, sherry, and hoisin in a Ziploc bag. Add steak and mix well. Remove excess air, seal, and marinate for at least 2 hours.
2) Thread steak into skewers and discard marinade.
3) For 5 minutes, cook on preheated 390° F or 199°C air fryer.
4) Serve and enjoy.

Nutrition Information:

- Calories per Serving: 130
- Carbs: 6.7g
- Protein: 14.7g
- Fat: 4.9g

Ginger, Garlic 'n Pork Dumplings

Servings per Recipe: 8

Cooking Time: 15

Ingredients:

- ¼ teaspoon crushed red pepper /1.25G
- ½ teaspoon sugar /2.5G
- 1 tablespoon chopped fresh ginger /15G
- 1 tablespoon chopped garlic /15G
- 1 teaspoon canola oil /5ML
- 1 teaspoon toasted sesame oil /5ML
- 18 dumpling wrappers
- 2 tablespoons rice vinegar /30ML
- 2 teaspoons soy sauce /10ML
- 4 cups bok choy, chopped
- 4 ounces ground pork /120G

Instructions:

1) Place a pan over heat, add the ginger and garlic sauté until fragrant. Add the ground pork and stir. Cook for 5 minutes.
2) Stir inside bok choy and crushed red pepper. Season with salt and pepper to taste. Allow to cool.
3) Place the meat mixture inside the middle of the dumpling wrappers. Fold the wrappers to seal the meat mixture in.

4) Place the book choy inside the grill pan.
5) Cook the dumplings in the air fryer at 330° F or 166°C for 15 minutes.
6) Meanwhile, prepare the dipping sauce by combining the remaining ingredients in a bowl.

Nutrition information:

- Calories per serving: 137
- Carbs: 16g
- Protein: 7g
- Fat: 5g

CPSIA information can be obtained
at www.ICGtesting.com
Printed in the USA
BVHW061939150621
609630BV00003B/403

9 781803 172446